Introduction to
Abbreviations Usec

G000122882

Welcome to the new 'Abbre

We have made some impro
popular booklet and I wanted to highlight these to you, ... ,
start using it.

This booklet can be used in two ways:
1. You can look up an abbreviation to get its meaning
2. You can find the right abbreviation by looking up the meaning.

We have removed the diagram section, as these are often used
variably in the clinical research environment and you are able to find
these in other reference books or on the Internet.

This booklet now has over 1750 abbreviations, collated by volunteers
working in clinical research. Compiling this booklet has been a
phenomenal task, and we are grateful to all contributors.

I hope that this booklet will prove useful to you, and if you have
suggestions for improving this and our other publications, please
contact us.

Helena Korjonen
Head of Information Services
www.icr-global.org

Abbreviation with meaning

ANDA	abbreviated new drug application (USA)
A on E	angina on exertion
A&A	alert and awake
A&E	accident and emergency
A&P	anterior and posterior
A&W	alive and well
A/K(A)	above knee (amputation)
A/W	able to work
AA	acute asthma; aortic aneurysm
AAA	abdominal aortic aneurysm
AAO	awake, alert and oriented
Ab	antibody
Abd	abdomen; abdominal
ABE	acute bacterial endocarditis
ABNM	American Board of Nuclear Medicine
ABPI	Association of the British Pharmaceutical Industry
ABR	absolute bed rest
ABS	absent
ABT	antibiotic therapy
AC	abdominal circumference; before food
ACC	advanced colorectal cancer
ACDM	Association of Clinical Data Management
ACE	angiotensin converting enzyme
ACIP	Advisory Committee on Immunisation Practices
ACJ	acromioclavicular joint
ACL	anterior cruciate ligament
ACLS	advance cardiac life support
ACM	alternative/complementary medicine
ACRP	Association of Clinical Research Professionals
ACRPI	Association of Clinical Research for the Pharmaceutical Industry now ICR
ACTH	adrenocorticotrophic hormone
AD	Alzheimer's disease

ADD	attention deficit disorder
ADE	adverse drug event or adverse device event
ADH	antidiuretic hormone
ADL	activities of daily living
ADME	absorption, distribution, metabolism and excretion
ADR	adverse drug reaction
AE	adverse event; air entry
AF	atrial fibrillation
AFB	acid fast bacillus
Ag	antigen
AHCA	American Healthcare Association
AHCPR	Agency for Health Care and Policy and Research
AI	aortic insufficiency
AICRC	Association of Independent Clinical Research Contractors
AID	absolute iron deficiency
AIDS	acquired immunodeficiency syndrome
AIMDD	active implantable medical devices
AJ	ankle jerk
AJCC	American Joint Committee on Cancer
AL	acute leukaemia
ALARA	as low as reasonably achievable
ALD	alcoholic liver disease
ALL	acute lymphocytic leukaemia
ALS	amyotrophic lateral sclerosis
ALT	alanine aminotransferase
AM	morning dose
AMA	against medical advice
AMBER	advanced multiple beam equilisation radiography
AMC	antibody-mediated cytotoxicity
AMI	acute myocardial infarction
AML	acute myeloid leukaemia
AMRC	Association of Medical Research Charities
ANF	antinuclear factor
Ang	angina
ANK	appointment not kept

A

B

Ank spond	ankylosing spondylitis
ANOVA	analysis of variance
Ant	anterior
AO	ankle oedema
AP	alkaline phosphatase; anteroposterior
APB	Association Pharmaceutique Belge (Belgium)
APC	advanced prostate cancer
APD	automated peritoneal dialysis
API	active pharmaceutical ingredient
APRN	advanced practice registered nurse
AR	adverse reaction; analytical standard of reagent purity; aortic regurgitation
ARC	AIDS-related complex
ARC	American Red Cross; Arthritis Research Campaign
ARCS	Association of Regulatory & Clinical Scientists (Australia)
ARD	acute respiratory disease
ARDS	acute respiratory distress syndrome
ARSAC	Administration of Radioactive Substances Advisory Committee
ART	artery/arterial
AS	aortic stenosis
ASAP	as soon as possible
ASD	atrial septal defect
AST	aspartate aminotransferase
AUC	area under the curve
AV	atrioventricular
AXR	abdominal X-ray

B/K(A)	below the knee (Amputation)
Ba	barium (eg, meal, enema)
BAC	benzalkonium chloride blood alcohol
BAL	British Anti-Lewisite (Dimercaprol)
BARQA	British Association of Research Quality Assurance
BBB	bundle branch block

BCC	basal cell carcinoma
BCG	bacillus almette-guérin vaccine (TB); ballistocardiogram (-graph)
BCR	British Comparative Ratio
BD/BID	twice a day
Be	Beryllium
BfArM	Bundesinstitut für Arzneimittel und Medizinprodukte (Federal Institute for Drugs and Medical Devices, Germany)
BGA	Bundesgesundheitsamt (Federal health office; former German public health agency)
BGW	Bundesinstitut für gesundheitlichen Verbraucher-schutz und Veterinärmedizin (Federal Institute for Health Protection of Consumers and Veterinary Medicine, Germany)
Bi	Bismuth
Bic	bicarbonate
BIH	benign intracranial hypertension
BIO	Biotechnology Industry Organization
BIPP	bismuth iodoform and paraffin paste
BIRA	British Institute of Regulatory Affairs (now TOPRA)
Bl/Bld	blood
BMR	basal metabolic rate
BN	batch number
BNF	British National Formulary
BNI	bladder neck incision
BNO	bowels not opened
BO	bowels open
BOE	breathlessness on exertion
BOO	bladder outflow obstruction
BP	blood pressure; boiling point; British Pharmacopoeia
BPC	British Pharmaceutical Codex
BPH	benign prostatic hypertrophy
BPI	Bundesverband der Pharmazeutischen Industrie EV (Germany)
BPM	beats per minute
Br	bromine
BrAPP	British Association of Pharmaceutical Physicians

The Institute of Clinical Research

	BS	bowel sounds; British Standard
	BSA	body surface area
	BSO	bilaterial salpingo-oophorectomy
	BSP	bromsulphthalein
	BTB	breakthrough bleed
	BUN	blood urea nitrogen
	Bx	biopsy
	C'	cervical spine
	c	with
	C&S	culture & sensitivity (to antibiotics)
	C/O	check out; complaining of
	C1	complement
	C1 C2 etc	1st, 2nd cervical vertebrae/nerves etc
	CA	competent authority (regulatory body charged with monitoring compliance with European Union member state national statutes and regulations); confidentiality agreement
	Ca	cancer/carcinoma; calcium
	Ca^{++}	calcium (ion)
	CAB	coronary artery bypass
	CABG	coronary artery bypass graft
	CAD	coronary artery disease
	CAI	chronic airways
	CAPD	continuous ambulatory peritoneal dialysis
	CAT	computer axial tomography
	CAV-H	continuous arteriovenous haemofiltration
	CAV-HD	continuous arteriovenous haemodialysis
	CBD	common bile duct
	CC	chief complaint
	CCF	congestive cardiac failure
	CCPRB	Comité Consultatif des Personnes participant à une recherché biomédiacle (French ethics committee)
	CCU	coronary care unit
	CD	controlled drug
	CDA	confidential disclosure agreement

CDER	Center for Drug Evaluation and Research (FDA)
CDH	congential dislocation of the hip
CDISC	Clinical Data Interchange Standards Consortium (formerly a DIA special interest group called the clinical data interchange standards committee)
CE-Mark	Conformité Européene
CEN	Comité Européen de Normalisation (European Committee for Standardization)
CF	consent form
cf	cystic fibrosis
CFR	code of federal regulations (FDA)
CGI	clinical global impressions (scale)
CGIC	clinical global impression of change
CH	chronic
CHF	congestive heart failure
CHMP	Committee for Medicinal Products for Human Use (formerly CPMP - Committee for Proprietary Medicinal Products)
CI	confidence interval (statistical term); Chief Investigator or Co-Investigator
CICU	cardiac intensive care unit
CIOMS	Council of International Organisations of Medical Sciences
CIU	clinical investigation unit
CK	creatinine kinase
CKF	chronic kidney disease
Claud	claudication
CLL	chronic lymphocytic leukaemia
C_{max}	maximum concentration (of drug)
CMC	chemistry, manufacturing and control
CME	continuing medical education
CMH	current medical history
C_{min}	minimum concentration (of drug)
CML	chronic myeloid leukaemia
CMR	client meeting report; centre for medical research
CMS	concerned member state
CMT	continuing medication and treatment
CMTX	chemotherapy treatment

The Institute of Clinical Research

CMV	cytomegalovirus
CNS	Clinical Nurse Specialist; central nervous system
CO	cardiac output
COAD	chronic obstructive airways disease
COC(P)	combined oral contraceptive (pill)
COD	cause of death
COLD	chronic obstructive lung disease
COMPASS	Computerised On-line Medicaid Pharmaceutical Analysis & Surveillance System
Consol	consolidation
Co-ord	co-ordination
COPD	chronic obstructive pulmonary disease
CORE	cardiovascular outcome and risk evaluation study
COREC	Central Office for Research Ethics Committees (UK)
COSTART	coding symbols for a thesaurus of adverse reaction terms
CP	chest pain
Cp	concentration of drug plasma
CPAP	continuous ambulatory peritoneal dialysis
CPK	creatinine phosphokinase
CPM	Clinical Project Manager
CPMP	Committee for Proprietary Medicinal Products (now known as CHMP – Committee for Medicinal Products for Human Use)
CPR	cardio-pulmonary resuscitation
CRA	Clinical Research Associate
CRC	clinical research centre
CRD	clinical research department
CRE	Clinical Research Executive
Creps	crepitations
CRF	case record form; chronic renal failure; clinical research facility
CRFCL	case report form correction logs
CRM	Clinical Research Manager
CRNA	Clinical Research Nurses Association
CRO	Contract Research Organisation
CRP	c-reactive protein
CS	caesarian section; current/cigarette smoker

CSF	cerebrospinal fluid
CSM	Committee on the Safety of Medicines; Clinical Study Manager
CSR	clinical study report
CT	computed tomography; clinical trial
CTA	Clinical Trial Administrator; Clinical Trial Agreement; Clinical Trial Authorisation
CTC	Clinical Trial Certificate
CTD	Clinical Trials Directive (EU); Common Technical Document (ICH)
CTE	clinical trial exemption
CTM	Clinical Trials Manager
CTMP	clinical trial on a marketed product
CTMS	clinical trial management system
CTR	Clinical Trial Report
CTS	carpal tunnel syndrome; clinical trial supplies
CTSM	Clinical Trial Supplies Manager
CTSU	clinical trials support unit
CTU	clinical trials unit
CTX	clinical trial exemption certificate (now incorporated into CTA)
CV	curriculum vitae
CVA	cerebro-vascular accident (stroke)
CVP	central venous pressure
CVS	cardiovascular system
Cx	cervical
Cx	circumflex artery
CXR	chest X-ray

D	discharge
D&C	dilatation and curettage
D&T	drugs and therapeutics
D&V	diarrhoea and vomiting
d/c	discharge; discontinue
DA	distension arthogram
da	iron deficiency anaemia

The Institute of Clinical Research

	DB	double blind
	DBMS	database management system
	DBP	diastolic blood pressure
	DC	diary card
	DCF	data collection form
	DCS	dynamic condylar screw
	DD	Department of Drugs (Sweden)
	dd	divided doses
	DDX	Doctors and Dentists Exemption Certificate
	DER	duodenal erosions
	DEXA	dual energy x-ray absorptiometry
	DGPharMed	Deutsche Gesellschaft für Pharmazeutische Medizin (German Society of Pharmaceutical Medicine)
	DH	Declaration of Helsinki; Department of Health (UK); drug history
	DHA	District Health Authority
	DHF	design history form
	DHS	dynamic hip screw
	DI	diabetes insipidus; donor insemination
	DIA	Drug Information Association
	DIC	disseminated intravascular coagulation
	Diff	differential blood count
	DIP(J)	distal interphalangeal (joint)
	Dis	distal
	DKA	diabetic ketoacidosis
	DLB	dementia
	DLE	discoid lupus erythematosus
	DLT	dose-limiting toxicity
	DM	diabetes mellitus
	DMC	data monitoring committee
	DMEC	data monitoring and ethics committee
	DMF	drug master file
	DNA	deoxyribonucleic acid; did not attend
	DNR	do not resuscitate
	DO	Doctor of Osteopathy
	DOA	dead on arrival

DOB	date of birth
DOCA	deoxycorticosterone acetate
DOE	dyspnoea on exertion
DPO	data protection officer
DQF(s)	data query form(s)
DRCGP	Diploma of the Royal College of General Practitioners
DRCOG	Diploma of the Royal College of Obstetrics & Gynaecology
DS	disseminated (multiple) sclerosis
DSA	digital subtraction angiography
DSH	deliberate self harm
DT's	delirium tremens
DTC	direct-to-consumer (drug advertising)
DTR	deep tendon reflex
DU	duodenal ulcer
DVT	deep vein thrombosis
DW	discussed with
D_X	diagnosis
DXT	deep x-ray therapy

E	erythrocytes; event/pre-existing condition
E/O	evidence of
EA	East/Southeast Asian (Burmese, Chinese, Japanese, Korean, Mongolian, Vietnamese); emergency admission; equivalent age
EAA	essential amino acids
EAB	ethical advisory board
EACA	epsilon-aminocaproic acid
EACR	European Association for Cancer Research
EANO	European Association for Neuro-Oncology
EAT	Edinburgh articulation test
EBL	estimated blood loss
EBM	evidence-based medicine; expressed breast milk
EBMT	European Group for Blood and Marrow Transplantation
EBRT	external beam radiation therapy
EBV	Epstein-Barr virus

EC	enterically coated; European Commission; Ethics Committee	
ECC	European Community Council	
ECF	extra-cellular fluid; extended family care	
ECG	electrocardiogram	
ECHO	echocardiography	
ECJ	European Court of Justice	
ECMO	extra-corporeal membrane oxygenation	
ECOG	Eastern Cooperative Oncology Group	
ECPHIN	European Community Pharmaceutical Products Information Network	
ECRF	electronic case report form	
ECRL	extensor carpi radialis longus	
e-CT	e-clinical trials	
ECT	electroconvulsive therapy	
ECT docs	electronic clinical trial documents	
e-CTD	electronic common technical document	
ED	effective dose; emergency department; erectile dysfunction; Executive Director; external diameter	
EDC	electronic data capture	
EDD	estimated date of discharge; estimated delivery date	
EDH	extradural haematoma	
EDI	electronic data interchange	
EDRF	endothelium-derived relaxing factor	
EDTA	ethylenediaminetraacetic acid	
EE	erosive oesophagitis	
EEA	European Economic Area	
EEC	European Economic Community, now EU	
EEG	electroencephalogram	
EENT	eye, ear, nose and throat	
EERS	electronic expense report system	
EET	established effective treatment	
EF	ejection fraction	
EFAD	essential fatty acid deficiency	
EFGCP	European Forum for Good Clinical Practice	
EFPIA	European Federation of Pharmaceutical Industries and Associations	

EFS	event free survival – time from diagnosis to defined events (eg relapse or death)
EFTA	European Free Trade Area/Association
EGD	oesophago-gastro duodenoscopy
EGF	epidermal growth factor
EHL	extensor hallucis longus
EHOR	European Health Outcomes Research
EIA	enzyme immuno assay
EIC	epidermal inclusion cyst
EIR	emotional insight research; establishment inspection report
EJ	external jugular
EKG	electrocardiogram (also known as ECG)
ELIZA	enzyme linked immunosorbent assay
ELSCS	elective lower segment caesarian section
EM	electron microscopy
EMC	encephalomyocarditis
EMEA	European Agency for the Evaluation of Medicinal Products
EMF	electromotive force
EMF	endomyocardial fibrosis; electromyogram (-graph)
EMLSCS	emergency lower segment caesarian section
eMR	electronic medical records
EMS	emergency medical system
EMT-B	Emergency Medical Technician – Basic
EMT-I	Emergency Medical Technician – Intermediate
EMT-P	Emergency Medical Technician – Paramedic
EMUO	early morning urine osmolarity (evaluating urine concentration)
EMWA	European Medical Writers Association
ENSG	European Neuroblastoma Study group
ENT	ear nose and throat
EOI	European Osteosarcoma Intergroup
EOM	extra-ocular muscles
EOMI	extra-ocular muscles intact
EORTC	European Organization for the Research and Treatment of Cancer
EOS	eosinophils

The Institute of Clinical Research

EP	early phase; electronic publishing; epilepsy; European Parliament	
EPA	Environmental Protection Agency	
EPH	edema proteinuria hypertension	
EPL	extensor pollicis longus	
EPO	erythropoietin	
EPRG	European Pharmacovigilance Research Group	
EPS	electrophysiological studies	
ER	electronic record; emergency room; essential requirements (EC); estrogen receptor	
ERB	ethical review board	
ERCP	endoscopic retrograde cholangio-pancreatography	
ERG	electroretinogram	
ERPC	evacuation of retained products of conception	
ERT	emergency response team	
ES	electrical simulation; epidural steroids; electronic signature	
ESI	epidural steroid injection	
ESICM	European Society of Intensive Care Medicine	
ESL	extracorporeal shockwave lithotripsy	
ESLD	end stage liver disease	
ESN	educationally subnormal	
ESO	European School of Oncology	
ESR	erythrocyte sedimentation rate	
ESRA	European Society of Regulatory Affairs (now TOPRA)	
ESRD	end stage renal disease	
ESRF	end stage renal failure	
ESSIR	European Society for Sexual Impotence Research	
ESTRO	European Society for Therapeutic Radiation and Oncology	
e-subs	electronic submissions	
ESWL	extracorporeal shockwave lithotripsy	
ET	endotracheal; endothelin; exercise test	
ETOH	ethanol or ethyl alcohol	
ETS	environmental tobacco smoke	
ETT	endotracheal tube; exercise tolerance test	
EU	European Union	
EU CTD	European Union Clinical Trials Directive	

A B C D **E** F G H I J K L M N O P Q R S T U V W X Y Z

EUA	examination under anaesthesia
EuCliD	European Clinical Development
EUCOMED	European Association of Medical Device Manufacturers
EudraCT	European Clinical Trials Database
EudraVigilance	European Database for Pharmacovigilance
EUS	endoscopic ultrasonography
EWCL	extended wear contact lenses
EWG	expert working group
EX	exclusion; flag used in laboratory reports to indicate an exclusion value according to the exclusion criteria set by sponsor
EX FIX	external fixation
EX LAP	exploratory laparotomy
EXP	expansion
EXT	extremities

F	Fahrenheit; female; finger
FA(b)	fluorescent antibody
FAQ	frequently asked questions
Farmindustria	Association of Italian Pharmaceutical Manufacturers
FB	finger breadths; foreign body
FBC	full blood count
FBS	fasting blood sugar
FD	forceps delivery; fully dilated
FDA	Food & Drug Administration (USA)
FDA 1571	IND application form (USA)
FDA 1572	statement of investigator form (USA)
FDA 1639	adverse event report form (USA)
FDA 356	NDA application form (USA)
FDP	flexor digitorum profundus
FDS	flexor digitorum superficialis
Fe def	iron deficiency
Fem Pop	femeropopliteal
FEV1	forced expiratory volume in one second
ff	force fluid

The Institute of Clinical Research

FFA	for further appointment; free fatty acids
FFP	fresh frozen plasma
FFPM	Fellow of the Faculty of Pharmaceutical Medicine (UK)
FH	family history; fundal height
FHR	foetal heart rate
FHS	foetal heart sounds
FHT	foetal heart tones
FiO_2	faction of inspired oxygen concentration
fl	fluids
FM	finger movement
FNA	fine needle aspiration
FNB	fine needle biopsy
FOB	faecal occult blood
FOS	full of stool / constipated
FP	freezing point
FP10	prescription
FPI	first patient in
FPO	first patient out
FRC	functional residual capacity
FRCP	Fellow of the Royal College of Physicians (UK)
FRCS	Fellow of the Royal College of Surgeons (UK)
FROM	full range of movement
FS	finger stick
FSH	follicle stimulating hormone
FT	full term
FTA	failed to attend
FTND	full term, normal delivery
FTT	failure to thrive
FU	follow up
FUB	functional uterine bleeding
FUO	fever of unknown origin
FVC	forced vital capacity
FW	foetal weight
FWB	full weight bearing
F_X	fracture
FYI	for your information

GA	general anaesthesia
G&D	growth & development
GAfREC	Governance Arrangements for Research Ethics Committees (UK)
GATT	General Agreement of Tariffs & Trade
GCP	good clinical practice
GCRP	good clinical research practice
GCS	Glasgow Coma Scale
GE	gastroenterology
GER	gastric erosions
GFR	glomerular filtration rate
GGT/γGT	gamma glutamyl transpeptidase
GH	growth hormone
GHTF	global harmonisation task force (medical devices)
GI(T)	gastro-intestinal (tract)
GLC	gas-liquid chromatography
GLP	good laboratory practice
Gls/Hb	glycosylated haemoglobin
GLU	glucose
GM	Geiger-Müller
GMP	good manufacturing practice
GORD	gastro oesophageal reflux disease
Grav	gravid (pregnant)
GTN	glyceral trinitrate
GTT	glucose tolerance test
GU	gastric ulcer; genito-urinary
GUM	genitor-urinary medicine
GUS	genitor-urinary system
Gyn	gynaecology
H&E	haematoxylin and eosin
H(O)CM	hypertrophic (obstructive) cardiomyopathy
H/A	headache
H/H	Henderson-Hasselbach equation (haemoglobin/hematocrit)
H°	null hypothesis (statistical term)

The Institute of Clinical Research

	H^1	alternative hypothesis (statistical term)
	H5N1	variant of Avian Flu
	HA	heart attack
	HA	hemaglutinin; hyperandrogenism
	HAD	3-Hydroxyacyl-COA Dehydrogenas (deficiency); hemadsorption (laboratory virus testing)
	HAF	hyperalimentation fluid
	HAI	Health Action International; hepatic activity index; hepatic arterial infusion
	HASCVD	hypertensive arteriosclerotic cardiovascular disease
	HASHD	hypertensive arteriosclerotic heart disease
	HAV, HBV	hepatitis A, B virus
	Hb	haemoglobin
	HB	heart block
	HBAIC	glycosylated haemoglobin
	HBI	hemi-body irradiation
	HBP	high blood pressure
	HCC	hepatocellular
	HCG	human chorionic gonadotrophin
	HCT	haematocrit
	HD	Hodgkin's disease
	HDL	high density lipoprotein
	HDU	high dependency unit
	HDx	haemodialysis
	HE	hepatic encephalopathy; hereditary elliptocytosis; hereditary erythrocytosis
	HEENT	head, eyes, ears, nose, throat
	Hep	hepatitis
	Hgb	haemoglobin
	HH	hiatus hernia
	HiB	haemophyllus influenza B
	HIPAA	Health Insurance Portability and Accountability Act (USA)
	HIV	human immunodeficiency virus
	HJR	hepatojugular reflex
	HLA	histocompatibility locus antigen
	HLA	human leukocyte antigens

HNPCC	hereditary nonpolyposis colorectal cancer
HO	House Officer
HPA	Health Protection Agency (UK)
HPAI	highly pathogenic form of avian influenza
HPC	hereditary prostate cancer; history of presenting condition/ complaint
HPI	history of presenting illness
HPLC	high performance liquid chromatography
HPV	human papilloma virus
HR	heart rate
HRPC	hormone refractory prostate cancer
HRT	hormone replacement therapy
HS	half strength; hand shaking; Hartman's solution; heart sounds; hemorrhagic septicaemia; hernial sac; herpes simplex
HSA	human serum albumin
HSM	hepatosplenomegaly
HSV	highly selective vagotomy; herpes simplex virus
HT;HTN	hypertension
HTLV	human lymphotopic virus, type III (aids agent, HIV)
Hx	history
HYST	hysterectomy
Hz	cycles per second (Hertz)

I	infusion
I+A	irrigation and aspiration
I+D	incision and drainage
I+R	insertion and removal
I&O; I/O; I+O	intake and output
i/c	with
IA	intra-arterial
IB	investigator's brochure
IBBBB	incomplete bilateral bundle branch block
IBD	inflammatory bowel disease
IBS	irritable bowel syndrome
IBW	ideal body weight

IC	intermittent claudication; informed consent; intermittent catheterisation	
ICAAC	Interscience Conference on Antimicrobial Agents and Chemotherapy	
ICD	International Classification of Diseases	
ICD9	International Classification of Diseases ninth edition	
ICF	intracellular fluid	
ICH	International Conference on Harmonisation	
ICR	Institute of Clinical Research	
ICS	intercostal space	
ICSI	intra cytoplasmic sperm injection	
ICU	intensive care unit	
ID	identity; infectious disease; internal diameter; inside diameter	
IDA	iron deficiency anaemia	
IDB	investigator's drug brochure	
IDDM	insulin dependent diabetes mellitus (Type 1)	
IDE study	investigational device exemption study (USA)	
IEC	Independent Ethics Committee	
IFAPP	International Federation of Associations of Pharmaceutical Physicians	
IFPMA	International Federation of Pharmaceutical Manufacturers Association	
IFU	instructions for use	
Ig	immunoglobulin	
IHD	incomplete heart block; ischaemic heart disease	
IKS	Interkantonale Kontrollstelle für Heilmittel (Switzerland)	
IL	interleukin	
ILBBB	incomplete left bundle branch block	
ILDL	intermediate low-density lipoprotein	
IM	intramuscular	
IMP	investigational materials plan; investigational medicinal product; impression/diagnosis	
IMPD	investigational medicinal product dossier	
IMV	intermittent mandatory ventilation	
IND	investigational new drug	
INF	inferior	

INR	international normalised ratio (clotting parameter)
INT	intestinal
INV	investigator
IP	intraperitoneal(ly); in-patient
IPPB	intermittent positive pressure breathing
IPPV	intermittent positive pressure ventilation
IQoL	individual quality of life questionnaire
IRB	independent review board; institutional review board
IRBBB	incomplete right bundle branch block
IRD	international registration document
IRDM	insulin resistant diabetes mellitus
IRMER	ionizing radiation medical exposure regulations
ISA	intrinsic sympathetic activity
ISCH	ischaemia
ISDN	isosorbide dinitrate
ISMN	isosorbide mononitrate
ISRCTN	international standard randomised controlled trial number
IT	intrathecal(ly)
ITP	idiopathic thrombocytopaenic purpura
ITT	insulin tolerance test; intention to treat
ITTP	intent to treat populations
ITU	intensive therapy unit
IUD	intrauterine device
IV	intravenous
IVC	intravenous cholangiogram; inferior vena cava
IVCD	intraventricular conduction defect
IVD	in-vitro diagnostics
IVDD	in-vitro diagnostic directive
IVF	in-vitro fertilisation
IVGTT	intravenous glucose tolerance test
IVI	intravenous infusion
IVP	intravenous pyelonephrogram
IVP/IVU	intravenous pyelography/urography
IVRS	interactive voice response system

The Institute of Clinical Research

°JCCLA	no jaundice, clubbing, cyanosis, lymphadenopathy, anaemia
J	joule
J, Jaun	jaundice
J; JT	joint
JCAHO	Joint Commission on Accreditation of Healthcare Organisations
JDM	juvenile diabetes mellitus
JDMS	juvenile dermatomyositis
JEV	Japanese encephalitis
JFS	Jewish Family Service
JJ	jaw jerk(s)
JME	juvenile myoclonic epilepsy
JODM	juvenile onset diabetes mellitus
JPMA	Japan Pharmaceutical Managers Association
JR	junctional rhythm
JRA	juvenile rheumatoid arthritis
JrBF	junior baby food
JRC	joint replacement centre
Jt	joint
JTPS	juvenile tropical pancreatitis syndrome
Juv	juvenile
JV	jugular vein
JVD	jugular venous distention
JVP	jugular venous pressure; jugular venous pulse
JVPT	jugular venous pulse trace
JW	Jehovah's Witness

K; K$^+$	potassium (ion)
KAT	katal (enzyme unit for transformation of one mole of substrate p. second under defined conditions)
KJ	knee jerk
KO	knocked out
KUB	kidney/ureters/bladder X ray
KW	Keith-Wagener ophthalmoscopic findings

_L	left
°LKKS/masses	no enlargement of liver, kidney, spleen or other palpable masses
L&D	labour and delivery
L&W	living and well
L/min	litres per minute
L1, L2 etc	1st, 2nd lumbar vertebrae/nerves etc
LA	local anaesthesia
Lab	laboratory
lac	laceration
LAD	left anterior descending; left anterior descending coronary artery; left axis deviation
LAE	left atrial enlargement
LAHB	left anterior hemi block
lam	laminectomy
Lap	laparotomy
Lap Chole	laparoscopic cholecystectomy
Lap Steri	laparoscopic sterilisation
lat	lateral
LATS	long-acting thyroid stimulator
LAVH	laparoscopic assisted vaginal hysterectomy
lax	laxative
LB	large bowel
LBBB	left bundle branch block
LBP	lower back pain
LBW	low birth weight
LCA	left coronary artery
LD	lethal dose
LD 50	median lethal dose
LDH	lactate dehydrogenase
LDL	low density lipoproteins
LE	lower extremities; lupus erythematosus
leuc	leukocytes
LF	low flap; low forceps
LFA	left front anterior
LFT	liver function tests; lung function tests

The Institute of Clinical Research

LH	lutenising hormone	
LHT	left hypertophia	
LICS	left intercostals space	
LIF	left iliac fossa; Läkemedelsindustriföreningen (The Swedish Association of the Pharmaceutical Industry)	
Lig	ligament	
LIH	left inguinal hernia	
Liq	liquid	
LKKS	liver; kidney right, left; spleen	
LL	lower lid	
LLE	left lower extremity	
LLG	left Lateral gaze	
LLL	left lower lobe	
LLQ	left lower quadrant	
LMD	family doctor	
LMM	lentigo maligna melanoma	
LMP	last menstrual period	
LOA	letter of agreement	
LOA	left occiput anterior	
LOC	loss of consciousness / level of consciousness	
LOM	left otitis media	
LOS	length of stay	
LOT	left occipital posterior	
LP	lumbar puncture	
LPI	last patient in	
LPN	Licensed Practice Nurse	
LPO	last patient out	
LREC	Local Research Ethics Committee	
LRQ	lower right quadrant	
LRTI	lower respiratory tract infection	
LS	locomotor system	
LSB	left sternal border	
LSCS	lower segment caesarean section	
LT	light touch	
LTH	prolactin (luteotrophic, lactogenic hormone)	
LUQ	left upper quadrant	

LVEDP	left ventricular and diastolic pressure
LVF	left ventricular failure
LVH	left ventricular hypertrophy
Lymphs	lymphocytes
Lytes	electrolytes
°masses	no enlargement of liver, kidney spleen or other palpable masses
M, C&S	microscopy, culture and sensitivity
m^2	square metres body surface
MA	Marketing Authorisation; Medical Advisor
MAA	Marketing Authorisation Application (EU)
MAC	Microbiology Advisory Committee
MAH	Marketing Authorisation Holder
MAIL	Medicines Act Information Letter
MAL	Medicines Act Leaflet
mane	morning
MANOVA	multivariate analysis of variance
MAOI	monoamine oxidase inhibitor
MC	metacarpal; Medicines Commission
MCA	Medicines Control Agency (now MHRA)
MCH	mean cell haemoglobin
MCHC	mean cell haemoglobin concentration
MCPJ	metacarpo-phalangeal joint
MCV	mean cell volume
MDA	medical device amendments
MDD	Medical Device Directive
MDR	medical device reporting
MDU	Medical Defence Union (UK)
Med	medial
MEDDEC	Medical Devices Guidance Document (for the EU Commission)
MedDRA	Medical Dictionary for Regulatory Activities
Meds	medicines
MEDWATCH	FDA safety information and AE reporting program
MEFA	Association of the Danish Pharmaceutical Industry

The Institute of Clinical Research

MEN	multiple endocrine neoplasia
MEP	Member of the European Parliament
mEq	milli-equivalent
MEST	maximal exercise stress test
METS	metastases
MHRA	Medicines and Healthcare Products Regulatory Agency
MHW	Ministry of Health and Welfare (Japan)
MI	myocardial infarction
MIBI	nuclear isotope scan (technetium / sestamibi)
MIC	minimum inhibitory concentration
MID	multi infarct dementia
MIMS	Monthly Index of Medical Specialties
mL	millilitre
MLD	minimum lethal dose
MLX	manufacturers licence exemption
mm	millimetre
mmHg	millimetre of mercury (measuring blood pressure)
mMOL	millimole (milliosmole, mosmol)
MMR	measles, mumps and rubella
MMSE	mini mental state examination
MND	motor neurone disease
MOA	mechanism of action
MOD	maturity onset diabetes
MOH	Ministry of Health
MOU	memorandum of understanding
MP	melting point
MPCC	medical pharmaceutical index
MR	mitral regurgitation
MRA	magnetic resonance angiography; mutual recognition agreement
MRC	Medical Research Council
MREC	Multicentre Research Ethics Committee
MRI	magnetic resonance imaging
MRSA	methicillin-resistant staphlococcus aureus
MS	member state; mitral stenosis; multiple sclerosis
MSH	melanophore-stimulating hormone

MSSU; MSU	midstream specimen of urine / midstream urine
MT	metatarsal
MTA	material transfer agreement
MTD	maximum tolerated dose
MTPJ	metatarsophalangeal joint
MTR	monitor's trip report
MUA	manipulation under anaesthetic
MUGA	multigated cardiac scan (nuclear isotope)
MVA	motor vehicle accident
MVD	microvascular decompression

N&M	night & morning
N&T	nose & throat
N or _N	normal
N&V; N/V	nausea and vomiting
N/n	overall size of sample
N/S	normal saline
NA	not applicable
Na; Na$^+$	sodium
NAD	no active disease; nothing abnormal discovered
NAI	no action indicated
NAS	new active substance
NBM	nil by mouth
NBP	non-evasive blood pressure
NCDM	Nordic Clinical Data Management (Association)
NCE	new chemical entity
NCR	no carbon required
NCRN	National Cancer Research Network (UK)
ND	not done
NDA	new drug application (USA)
NDAB	National Drugs Advisory Board (Ireland)
NED	no evidence of recurrent disease
NEFA	non-esterified fatty acids
NEFARMA	Dutch Association of the Innovative Pharmaceutical Industry
NER	no evidence of recurrence

NFA	no further appointment
NG	naso-gastric
NH MRC	National Health and Research Council (Australia)
NHS	National Health Service (UK)
NICU	neonatal intensive care unit
NIDDM	non-insulin dependent diabetes mellitus (Type 2)
NIH	National Institute of Health (USA)
NK	not known
NKA	no known allergies
NME	new molecular entity
NMR	nuclear magnetic resonance (imaging)
Nocté	nightly
NOEL	no observable effect level
NOF	neck of femur
NOH	neck of humerus
NPL	National Physical Laboratory (UK)
NPN	non-protein nitrogen
NPO	nothing by mouth
NPSA	National Patient Safety Agency
NRM	no regular medicines
NS	non smoker; not significant
NSAID	non-steroidal anti-inflammatory drug
NSCLC	non-small cell lung carcinoma
NSTS	NHS Strategic Tracing Service (UK)
NSU	non-specific urethritis
NTP	normal temperature pressure
NUD	non-ulcer dyspepsia

°	absent, eg °BS = absence of bowel sounds
o	by mouth
O/A	on admission
O/E	on examination
OA	osteoarthritis
OBGYN	obstetrics & gynaecology
Obs Gyn	obstetrics and gynaecology

OCD	obsessive compulsive disorder
OCP	oral contraceptive pill
OCT	orthotopic cardiac transplant
OD	once a day; overdose; outside diameter
OGD	oesophago-gastro-duodenoscopy
OH	occupational health
OHS	Occupational Health Service (UK)
OM	once daily in the morning
ON	once daily at night
ONS	Office of National Statistics (UK)
OOH	out of hours
OPA	outpatient's appointment
OPD	outpatients department
Or	both eyes
OR	operating room
ORIF	open reduction & internal fixation
ORL	otorhinolaryngology
Os	left eye
OSAS	obstructive sleep apnoea syndrome
OT	occupational therapy; operating theatre
OTC	over the counter
Ou	right eye

P&A	percussion and auscultation
PA	pascal
PA; P-A	posterioanterior
PAC	premature atrial, auricular contraction
$PaCO_2$	arterial carbon dioxide tension pressure – arterial CO_2
PACU	post anaesthesia care unit
Paeds	paediatrics
PAF	paroxysmal atrial fibrillation; platelet aggregating factor
Palp	palpate, palpated, palpable
PAN	polyarteritis nodosa
PaO_2	arterial oxygen pressure
Pap	Papanicolaou test (pap smear)

The Institute of Clinical Research

PAP	pulmonary artery pressure
PAR	post-approval research
Para	prior births; paraplegic
PARU	post anaesthesia recovery unit
PAS	patient administration system; periodic acid Schiff reagent; pulmonary artery systolic pressure
PAT	paroxysmal atrial tachycardia; pregnancy at term
Path	pathology
PAWP	pulmonary artery wedge pressure
PB	peripheral blood
Pb	lead
PBC	primary biliary cirrhosis
PBI	protein bound iodine
PC; P/C	presenting complaint
PCA	patient controlled analgesia
PCA	patient controlled angina
PCC	poison control centre
PCG	phonocardiogram
PCL	posterior cruciate ligament
PCN	percutaneous nephrolithotomy
PCO_2	carbon dioxide concentration
PCP	pneumocystis carinii pneumonia
PCT	Primary Care Trust (UK)
PCV	packed cell volume
PD	Parkinson's disease; papillary distance; peritoneal dialysis; pharmacodynamics; Pick's disease
PDA	patent ductus arteriosus ; personal digital assistant
PDF	portable document format
Pdr	powder
PE	physical examination
PE	pulmonary embolism
PEEP	positive and expiratory pressure
PEF(R)	peak expiratory flow (rate)
PEG	pneumoencephalogram
PEN	penicillin
PERLA	pupils equal and reactive to light and accommodation

PEP POTENTIAL END POINT

PESA	percutaneous epidimal sperm aspiration
PET	positron emission tomography; pre-eclampsic toxaemia
PF	peak flow
PFC	positive foetal circulation
PFTs	pulmonary function tests
PH	past history
pH	measure of acidity/alkalinity
Pharm	pharmacy
Phys	physical or physiology
PI	Principal Investigator; package insert; present illness; pulmonary insufficiency
PIAG	patient information advisory group
PICA	posterior inferior coronary artery
PICU	paediatric intensive care unit
PID	pelvic inflammatory disease
PIL	patient information leaflet
PIPA	Pharmaceutical Information & Pharmacovigilance Association
PIP(J)	proximal interphalangeal (joint)
PIS	patient information sheet
Pit	pitocin
PK	pharmacokinetics
PKU	phenylketonuria
PL	product licence
PLA	product licence application
Plac	placenta
plant	plantar (reflexes)
Plts	platelets
PM	evening dose; petit mal; post-mortem; evening dose
PMA	Pharmaceutical Manufacturers' Association (USA); post-marketing approval
PMH	past medical history
PMI	point of maximum impulse
PMN	polymorphonuclear (leukocytes)
PMO	post-menopausal osteoporosis
PMS	post-marketing surveillance
PMSG	pregnant mare's serum gonadotrophin

PMT	pre-menstural tension
Pn	percussion
PND	paroxysmal nocturnal dyspnoea
Pneu	pheumo or pneumonia
PNI	peripheral nerve injury
Pnx	pneumothorax
po	by mouth (per os)
P0,AB1	no births, one abortion
PO_2	oxygen pressure (or tension)
POC	product of conception
pod	postoperative day
Poly	polymorphonuclear leucocytes
POM	prescription only medicine
POP	plaster of paris
Pos	positive
Post	posterior
PP	peripheral pulses; pinprick
Pp	post partum; post prandial
PPBS	post prandial blood sugar
PPD	purified protein derivative
PPH	post partum haemorrhage
PPI	patient pack insert
PPM	parts per million
PPPG	post prandial plasma glucose
PR	per rectum; pulse rate
PR interval	an ECG interval
PRA	plasma rennin activity
PRN	taken as required
prox	proximal
PS	plastic surgery
PS	pulmonary stenosis
PSH	past surgical history
PSI	Statisticians in the Pharmaceutical Industry (UK)
Psi	pounds per square inch
PSMA	progressive spinal muscular atrophy
PSVT	paroxysmal supraventricular tachycardia

PT	prothrombin time
PTA	prior to admission
PTC	percutaneous transhepatic cholangiography
PTCA	percutaneous coronary angioplasty
PTH	parathyroid hormone
PTHC	percutaneous transhepatic cholangiogram
PTT	partial thromboplastin time
PU	passed urine ; peptic ulcer
PUD	peptic ulcer disease
PUJ	pelviureteric junction
PUO	pyrexia of unknown origin
PV	per vagina
PVC	premature ventricular contraction
PVR	peripheral vascular resistance
PVS	peripheral vascular system
pwb	partial weight bearing
Px	past history
Px	pneumothorax
Px	prognosis

Q	every
Q2H	every 2 hours
Q3H	every 3 hours
QA(U)	quality assurance (unit)
QAC	before every meal
QALE	quality-adjusted life expectancy
QALY	quality-adjusted life year
QAM	each morning
QAS	quality-adjusted survival
QC	quality control
QCD	quality control department
QDS; QID	four times a day
QE	quinidine effect
QED	quick and early diagnosis; every day
QHS	at each bedtime

QL	quality of life
QLI	quality of life index
QLS	quality of life score
QMS	quality management system
QOL	quality of life
QOLQ	quality of life questionnaire
QP	Qualified Person (responsible for the final dispatch of study drugs)
QPM	each evening
QPOS	quality point of service
QQH	every four hours
QWB	quality of well-being

_R	right
R&D	research and development
RA	regional anaesthetic; routine admission; rheumatoid arthritis
RADAR	risk assessment of drugs – analysis and response
RAST	radioallergosorbent test
RBBB	right bundle branch block
RBC	red blood cell (corpuscle)
RBE	relative biological effectiveness
RCA	right coronary artery
RCT	randomised clinical trial
RDE	remote data entry
RDS	respiratory distress syndrome
REC	Research Ethics Committee
rect	rectally
ref	reflexes
reg	regular
REM	rapid eye movement
RF	renal failure
RH	relative humidity
Rh	Rhesus factor
RhA	rheumatoid arthritis
RHD	rheumatic heart disease

RhF	rheumatic fever/factor
RIA	radioimmunoassay
RICP	raised intracranial pressure
RIF	right iliac fossa
RIH	right inguinal hernia
RLQ	right lower quadrant (abdominal)
RN	Registered Nurse (UK)
RNA	ribonucleic acid
ROM	range of motion
ROS	review of systems
RP	radial pulse
RPF	renal plasma flow
RPO	Radiation Protection Officer
RQ	respiratory quotient
RR	respiratory rate
RS	respiratory system
RSDS	reflex sympathetic dystrophy syndrome
RT	radiotherapy; reaction time (neurophysiology)
RTA	road traffic accident
RTI	respiratory tract infection
RUJ	radioulnar joint
RUQ	right upper quadrant
RVF	right ventricular failure
Rx	drug history; prescribe; prescription; treatment

S&O	salpingo oophorectomy
S&C	sclerae and conjunctive
S&E	screening and evaluation; sugar and acetone
S&H	speech and hearing
S&I	supervision and interpretation
S&M	surveillance and maintenance
S&S	signs and symptoms
S DATA	self-report data
S/B	seen by
S/P	status post

The Institute of Clinical Research

S1, S2 etc	1st, 2nd, sacral vertebrae/nerves etc
S1/S2/S3/S4	heart sounds
S-A	sino-artrial
SAA	synthetic amino acid
SAD	seasonal affective disorder
SADE	serious adverse device event
S-ADHD	secondary adhd
SAE	serious adverse event
SAH	sub-arachnoid haemorrhage
S-Anill	secondary acute non lymphoid leukemia
SaO_2	oxygen saturation
SAR	serious adverse reaction
SBE	subacute bacterial endocarditis
SBFT	small bowel follow through
SBP	systolic blood pressure
SBS	small bowel movement
SC	static compliance; subcutaneous
SCC	squamous cell carcinoma
SCJ	sternoclavicular joint
SCM	sternocleidomastoid
SCr	serum creatinine
SD	standard deviation
SDAT	senile dementia Alzheimer type
SDH	sub-dural haematoma
SDV	source data/document verification
SE	substantially equivalent; standard error (statistical term)
SEM	standard error of mean; systolic ejection murmer
Sen	sensation
SF	site file
SG	Swan-Ganz
SGA	small for gestational age
SGGT	serum gamma-glutamyl transpeptidase
SGOT	serum glutamic-oxaloacetic transaminase
SGPT	serum glutamic-pyruvic transaminase
SH	social history
SHO	Senior House Officer

Sl	sterilization
SIADH	syndrome of inappropriate ADH secretion
Sig	write-on label
SIJ	sacro-illiac joint
SIMV	synchronous intermittent mandatory ventilation
SIRI	aalivary immunoreactive insulin
SL	sub-lingual
SLE	systemic lupus erythematosus
SMA	superior mesenteric artery
SME	significant medical event
SMO	Site Management Organization
SmPC	summary of product characteristics
SNIP	Syndicat National de l'Industrie Pharmaceutique (France)
SO	sutures out
SOA	statement of agreement
SOAP	subjective, objective, assessment and plans
SOB	shortness of breath
SOBAR	shortness of breath at rest
SOBOE	shortness of breath on exertion
Solid CO_2	dry ice
SOP(s)	standard operating procedure(s)
SOS	if necessary
Spl	spleen
SPM	Society of Pharmaceutical Medicine
SpR	specialist registrar
SQ	subcutaneous
SR	Senior Registrar; sinus rhythm
SSA	site-specific approval; Site-Specific Assessor
SSC	Study Site Coordinator
SSCT	Swedish Society for Clinical Trials
SSFA	Società di Scienze Farmacologiche Applicate (Italy)
SSS	sick sinus syndrome
stat	immediately
SUA	serious unexpected adverse event
sublux	subluxation
SUD	sudden unexpected death

SUE	serious unexpected event
sup	superior; supine
SUSAR	suspected unexpected serious adverse reaction
SV	stroke volume
SVC	superior vena cava
SVD	spontaneous vaginal delivery
SVT	supraventricular tachycardia
SW	social worker
Sx	symptoms
SXR	skull x-ray

3TC	lamivudine (Epivir)
T	tension ; testicles ; thymine ; trace ; temperature ; testosterone; thoracic
T-	decreased intraocular tension
T&N	tension & nervousness; tingling & numbness
T (0)	oral temperature
T cell	small lymphocyte
T max	time to maximum
t test	student t-test
T&E	testing and evaluation; trial and error; training and evaluation
T+	increased intraocular tension
T°	temperature
T•	one tablet, once a day
T••	two tablets, once a day
T1	tricuspid first sound
T1, T2 etc	1st, 2nd, thoracic vertebrae/nerves etc
T1/2	half life (of a drug)
T2	triscuid second sound
T3	tri-iodothyronine
T3/4 ind	triiodothyronine to thyroxine index
T4	CD4 (helper inducer cells); thyroxine
TA	temperature auxiliary ; temporal arteritis ; tendon achilles ; therapeutic abortion; traffic accident; truncus arterious

TAA	therapeutic activities aid; tumour-associated antigen (antibodies)
TAB	tablet; triple antibiotic
TAC	tetracine, adrenalin® and cocaine; total allergen content
TAH	transabdominal hysterectomy
TAP	total adipose fat; tumour activated pro-drug; turnaround time
TAPVC	total anomalous pulmonary venous connection
TAPVD	total anomalous pulmonary venous drainage
TAPVR	total anomalous pulmonary venous return
TAR	treatment administration report/record; treatment authorisation request
TAS	therapeutic activities specialist; typical absence seizures
TAUC	target area under the curve
TB	tapes for the blind; total bilirubin; total bilirubin; tuberculosis
TBA	to be absorbed; to be added; to be administered; to be admitted; to be announced; to be arranged; to be assessed
TBA	total body (surface) area
TBC	to be cancelled; total blood cholesterol; total body clearance; tuberculosis
TBD	to be determined
TBE	tick-borne encephalitis
TBF	total body fat
TBG	thyroxine blood globulin
TBI	total body irradiation; traumatic brain injury
TBK	total body potassium
TBMg	total body magnesium
TBN	total body nitrogen
TBNa	total body sodium
TBP	total body phosphorous
TBP	total body protein
TBR	total bed rest
TBS	table spoon; to be seen; total serum bilirubin
TBSA	total body surface area
TBT	tolbutamid test
TBV	total blood volume
TBW	total body water

TC		team conference; telephone call; terminal cancer; testicular cancer; throat culture; trachealcollar; thoracic circumference; tissue culture; total cholesterol
TCA		tricyclic antidepressant
TCA		tumour chemosensitivity assay
TCE		total colon examination
TCI		to come in
TCID		tissue culture infected dose
TCM		tissue culture media
TCM		traditional Chinese medicine
TCM		transcutaneous monitor
TCMH		tumour-direct cell-mediated hypersensitivity
TCR		t-cell receptor
TCT		triple combination tablet
TCU		transitional care unit
TD		temporary disability; terminal device; tidal volume; tolerance dose; total disability; treatment discontinued; treatment discontinued
TDD		telephone device for the deaf
TDF		total dietary fibre
TDI		tolerable daily intake
TDM		therapeutic drug monitoring
TDN		total digestible nutrients
TdP		torsades de pointes
TdR		thymidine
TDS		three times a day
TDx®		flourescence polarisation immunoassay
TE		terminal extension; toothaches; total exploratory time; total exploratory time
TeBG		testosterone binding globulin
TEC		toxic escherichia coli
TED		thromboembolic disease
TEDS		thromboembolic disease stockings
TEE		total energy expended
TEI		total episode of illness
TEL		telephone

TEM	transmission electron microscopy
TEMP	temperature temporal tension
temp	temperature
TENS	transcutaneous nerve stimulation
TEQ	toxic equivalence
TER	total energy requirement
TERT	tertiary
TES	testicular extraction of sperm; treatment emergent symptoms
TESE	testicular sperm extraction
TESS	treatment emergent symptom scale
TET	treadmill exercise test
TF	tube feeding
TFA	trans fatty acids
TFBC	The Family Birthing Centre
TFR	total fertility rate
TFT	thyroid function test
TG	triglycerides
Tg	thyroglobulin
TGA	third generation anti-depressant
TGF	transforming growth factor
TH	thyroid hormone; total hysterectomy
THBI	thyroid hormone binding index
THBR	thryoid hormone binding ratio
THC	thigh circumference
THP	take home packs
THR	target heart rate; total hip replacement; training heart rate
THTV	therapeutic home trial visit
TIA	transient ischaemic attack (cerebral)
tib/fib	tibula/fibula
TIBC	total iron binding capacity
TICU	thoracic intensive care unit; trauma intensive care unit
TID	three times a day
TIND	treatment investigational new drug
TISS	therapeutic intervention scoring system
TK	toxicokinetics
TKR	total knee replacement

The Institute of Clinical Research

TL	thallium; team leader; terminal latency; trial leave
TLC	temporal lobe epilepsy; tender loving care; thin layer chromatography; total lung capacity
TLV	total lung volume
Tm	maximal renal tubular clearance
TM	trade mark; tropical medicine; tumour
TMA	trained medication aid
TMAS	Taylor Manifest Anxiety Scale
T_{max}	the time after dosing when Cmax occurs; time to maximum
TMET	treadmill exercise test
TMF	trial master file
TMG	Trial Management Group
TMJ	temporomandibular joint
TMM	total muscle mass
TMST	treadmill stress test
TNA	total nutrient add mixture
TNB	term newborn
TND	term normal delivery
TNF	tumour necrosis factor
TNG	nitroglycerin
TO	transfer out; total obstruction
TOB	tobacco
TOC	table of contents
TOH	throughout hospitalisation
TOM	therapeutic outcomes monitoring; tomorrow
TOP	termination of pregnancy
top	topical
TOPRA	The Organisation for Professionals in Regulatory Affairs
TOPV	trialvalent oral polio vaccine
TORC	test of reading comprehension
TOWL	test of written language
TP	thought process; treating physician; total protein
TPC	target plasma concentration; total patient care
TPHA	treponema pallidum haemagglutination assay
TPM	temporary pacemaker
TPN	total parenteral nutrition

TPO	trial prescription order
TPR	temperature, pulse, respiration
TPR	total peripheral resistance
TPT	treadmill performance test
TR	therapeutic respiration; time to repeat; trace; transplant recipients; treatment; tumour registry; tremor; tricuspid incompetence
trach	trachea(l)
TRAM	treatment response assessment method
TRBC	total red blood cells
TRD	treatment related death
TRD	treatment resistant depression
TRM	transplant related mortality; treatment related mortality
TrPs	trigger points
TRPT	transplant
TRS	therapeutic recreation specialist
TS	Tay-Sachs (disease); test solution; trauma score; tricuspid stenosis; triple strength; Turner's syndrome; telomerase; temperature sensitive; throat swab; Tourette's syndrome; transsexual; tuberous sclerosis
Ts	t suppressor cell
TSA	type-specific antibody; total shoulder arthroplasty; tumour specific antigen
TSAb	thyroid stimulating antibodies
TSAS	total severity assessment score
TSB	total serum bilirubin
TSC	trial steering committee
TSE	targeted systemic exposure ; testicular self-examination; total skin examination
TSGs	tumour suppressor genes
TSH	thyroid stimulating hormone (thyrotropin)
TSI	thyroid stimulating immunoglobulin
TSP	total serum protein
TSS	total serum solids; toxic shock syndrome
TST	treadmill stress test
TT	Test Tape®; thrombin time; transit time; twitch tension
TT	twitch tension

TT ••	two tablets, twice a day
TT•	one tablet, twice a day
TT4	total thyoxine
TTAs; TTOs	to take away/to take out ie medications to take home
TTDP	time to disease progression
TTM	total tumour mass
TTO	transtracheal oxygen
TTO	tea tree oil
TTP	tender to pressure; time to pregnancy; time to tumour progression
TTS	through the skin
TTT	tolbutamide tolerance test
TTV	transfusion transmitted virus
TUF	total ultra filtration
TUG	total urinary gonadatropin
TUN	total urinary nitrogen
TURP	trans-urethral resection of prostate
TURT	trans-urethral resection of tumour
TV	transvenous; trial visit; trial volume; tricuspid valve
TVD	triple vessel disease
TVF	tactile vocal fremitus
TVH	transvaginal hysterectomy
TVI	time velocity integral
TVR	tricuspid valve replacement
TW	tap water; test weight; t-wave
TWD	total white and differential count
TWG	total weight gain
Tx	therapist/therapy; traction ; transcription ; transfuse ; transplant
TX	treatment

U&E	urea and electrolytes
UA	unavailable
UC	ulcerative colitis
UGS	uro-genital system

UID	once a day
UKCRC	UK Clinical Research Collaboration
UKCRN	UK Clinical Research Network
Ukn	unknown
URTI	upper respiratory tract infection
US; USS	ultrasound scan
USGB	ultrasound gall bladder
UTI	urinary tract infection
UV	ultraviolet
V	vomiting
V&P	vagotomy and pyloroplasty
V/Q	ventilation/perfusion
VA	visual acuity
VAD	vincristine adriblastine dexamethasone
VAERS	vaccine adverse event reporting system (FDA)
vag	vaginally
VAI	voluntary action indicated
VAMC	Veterans Affairs Medical Centre
VAMP	vincristine adriblastine methylprednisone
VAS	visual analogue scale
VATS	video assisted thoracoscopic surgery
VAX	vaccine
VBAC	vaginal birth after caesarean
VBG	venous blood gas
VBI	vertebrobasilar insufficiency
VC	vital capacity; vocal chord
vCJD	variant Creutzfeldt-Jakob disease
VCUG	voiding cysto-urethrogram
VD	vaginal delivery; vascular dementia; venereal disease
VDRL	venereal diseases research laboratory
VE	vaginal examination
VEB	ventricular ectopic beat
VEF	ventricular ejection fraction (test lung function)
VEN	venous

The Institute of Clinical Research

VF	ventricular fibrillation
VF	vocal fremitus
vib	vibration
VID	volunteer information document
VIP	vasoactive intestinal peptide
Vis Mem	visual memory
VLDL	very low density lipoprotein
VM	vastus medialis
VMA	vanilmandelic acid; vanillylmandelic acid
VMD	Veterinary Medical Doctor
VOC	voice of the customer; volatile organic compound
VOE	voice of the employee
VP	ventriculoperitoneal; verruca pedis
VPA	valproic acid
VRE	vancomycin resistant enterococci
VS	vital signs
VSD	ventricular septal defect
VSS	vital signs stable
VT	ventricular tachycardia
VTE	venous thromboembolic events
VV	varicose veins
VW	vessel wall
VWF	Von Willebrand Factor

WR	ward round
WBC	white blood corpuscle
WCC	white cell count (diff = differential)
WDWN	well developed; well nourished
WHO	World Health Organization
WNL	within normal limits
WPW	Wolff-Parkinson-White (syndrome)

X&D	examination and diagnosis
X match	cross match (blood transfusion)
XR	x-ray
Y/O	years old
Z/D	zero defects
Z-DNA	zig zag deoxyribonucleic acid
ZE syndrome	Zollinger-Ellison syndrome
Z-ESR	zeta erythrocyte sedimentation rate
Z-TSP	zephiran trisodium phosphate

The Institute of Clinical Research

A
B
C
D
E
F
G
H
I
J
K
L
M
N
O
P
Q
R
S
T
U
V
W
X
Y

Find an abbreviation

3-Hydroxyacyl-COA Dehydrogenas (deficiency)	HAD
alternative hypothesis (statistical term)	H1
abbreviated new drug application (USA)	ANDA
abdomen, abdominal	Abd
abdominal aortic aneurysm	AAA
abdominal circumference	AC
abdominal X-ray	AXR
able to work	A/W
above knee (amputation)	A/K(A)
absent	ABS
absent, eg °BS = absence of bowel sounds	°
absolute bed rest	ABR
absolute iron deficiency	AID
absorption, distribution, metabolism and excretion	ADME
accident and emergency	A&E
acid fast bacillus	AFB
acquired immunodeficiency syndrome	AIDS
acromioclavicular joint	ACJ
active implantable medical devices	AIMDD
active pharmaceutical ingredient	API
activities of daily living	ADL
acute asthma	AA
acute bacterial endocarditis	ABE
acute leukaemia	AL
acute lymphocytic leukaemia	ALL
acute myeloid leukaemia	AML
acute myocardial infarction	AMI
acute respiratory disease	ARD
acute respiratory distress syndrome	ARDS
Administration of Radioactive Substances Advisory Committee	ARSAC
adrenocorticotrophic hormone	ACTH
advance cardiac life support	ACLS
advanced colorectal cancer	ACC

advanced multiple beam equilisation radiography	AMBER
advanced practice registered nurse	APRN
advanced prostate cancer	APC
adverse drug event or adverse device event	ADE
adverse drug reaction	ADR
adverse event	AE
adverse event report form (USA)	FDA
adverse reaction	AR
Advisory Committee on Immunisation Practices	ACIP
against medical advice	AMA
Agency for Health Care and Policy and Research	AHCPR
AIDS-related complex	ARC
air entry	AE
alanine aminotransferase	ALT
alcoholic liver disease	ALD
alert and awake	A&A
alive and well	A&W
alkaline phosphatase	AP
alternative/complementary medicine	ACM
Alzheimer's disease	AD
American Board of Nuclear Medicine	ABNM
American Healthcare Association	AHCA
American Joint Committee on Cancer	AJCC
American Red Cross	ARC
amyotrophic lateral sclerosis	ALS
an ECG interval	PR interval
analysis of variance	ANOVA
analytical standard of reagent purity	AR
angina	Ang
angina on exertion	A on E
angiotensin converting enzyme	ACE
ankle jerk	AJ
ankle oedema	AO
ankylosing spondylitis	Ank spond
anterior	Ant

The Institute of Clinical Research

A

anterior and posterior	A&P
anterior cruciate ligament	ACL
anteroposterior	AP
antibiotic therapy	ABT
antibody	Ab
antibody-mediated cytotoxicity	AMC
antidiuretic hormone	ADH
antigen	Ag
antinuclear factor	ANF
aortic aneurysm	AA
aortic insufficiency	AI
aortic regurgitation	AR
aortic stenosis	AS
appointment not kept	ANK
area under the curve	AUC
arterial carbon dioxide tension pressure – arterial CO_2	$PaCO_2$
arterial oxygen pressure	PaO_2
artery/arterial	ART
as low as reasonably achievable	ALARA
as soon as possible	ASAP
aspartate aminotransferase	AST
Association for Information Officers in the Pharmaceutical Industry	AIOPI
Association of Clinical Data Management	ACDM
Association of Clinical Research for the Pharmaceutical Industry now ICR	ACRPI
Association of Independent Clinical Research Contractors	AICRC
Association of Italian Pharmaceutical Manufacturers	Farmindustria
Association of Medical Research Charities	AMRC
Association of Regulatory & Clinical Scientists (Australia)	ARCS
Association of the British Pharmaceutical Industry	ABPI
Association of the Danish Pharmaceutical Industry	MEFA
Association Pharmaceutique Belge (Belgium)	APB
at each bedtime	QHS
atrial fibrillation	AF
atrial septal defect	ASD

atrioventricular	AV
attention deficit disorder	ADD
automated peritoneal dialysis	APD
awake, alert and oriented	AAO

bacillus almette-guérin vaccine (TB)	BCG
ballistocardiogram (-graph)	BCG
barium (eg meal, enema)	Ba
basal cell carcinoma	BCC
basal metabolic rate	BMR
batch number	BN
beats per minute	BPM
before every meal	QAC
before food	AC
below the knee (amputation)	B/K(A)
benign intracranial hypertension	BIH
benign prostatic hypertrophy	BPH
benzalkonium chloride blood alcohol	BAC
Beryllium	Be
bicarbonate	Bic
bilaterial salpingo-oophorectomy	BSO
biopsy	Bx
Biotechnology Industry Organization	BIO
Bismuth (chemical symbol)	Bi
bismuth iodoform and paraffin paste	BIPP
bladder neck incision	BNI
bladder outflow obstruction	BOO
blood	Bl; Bld
blood pressure	BP
blood urea nitrogen	BUN
body surface area	BSA
boiling point	BP
both eyes	Or
bowel sounds	BS

The Institute of Clinical Research

B

C

The Institute of Clinical Research

Council of International Organisations of Medical Sciences	....	CIOMS
c-reactive protein	....	CRP
creatinine kinase	....	CK
creatinine phosphokinase	....	CPK
crepitations	....	Creps
cross match (blood transfusion)	....	X match
culture & sensitivity (to antibiotics)	....	C&S
current medical history	....	CMH
current/cigarette smoker	....	CS
curriculum vitae	....	CV
cycles per second (Hertz)	....	Hz
cystic fibrosis	....	cf
cytomegalovirus	....	CMV
data collection form	....	DCF
data monitoring and ethics committee	....	DMEC
data monitoring committee	....	DMC
data protection officer	....	DPO
data query form(s)	....	DQF(s)
database management system	....	DBMS
date of birth	....	DOB
dead on arrival	....	DOA
declaration of elsinki (also DoH)	....	DH
decreased intraocular tension	....	T-
deep tendon reflex	....	DTR
deep vein thrombosis	....	DVT
deep x-ray therapy	....	DXT
deliberate self harm	....	DSH
delirium tremens	....	DT's
dementia	....	DLB
deoxycorticosterone acetate	....	DOCA
deoxyribonucleic acid	....	DNA
Department of Drugs (Sweden)	....	DD
Department of Health	....	DH

The
Institute
of
Clinical
Research

E

The Institute of Clinical Research

foetal heart sounds . . . . FHS

foetal heart tones. . . . . FHT

foetal weight. . . . . FW

follicle stimulating hormone . . . . FSH

follow up . . . . FU

following a PL, response from MCA requesting more information . . . . . . letter

Food & Drug Administration (USA) . . . . FDA

Bundesinstitut für Arzneimittel und Medizinprodukte
   (Federal Institute for Drugs and Medical Devices, Germany) . . . . BfArM

for further appointment . . . . .FFA

for your information . . . . FYI

force fluid . . . . ff

forced expiratory volume in one second FEV1

forced vital capacity . . . . FVC

forceps delivery . . . . FD

foreign body . . . . .FB

Bundesgesundheitsamt (Federal health office;
   former German public health agency) . . . . BGA

four times a day . . . . .QDS; QID

fracture . . . . .FX

free fatty acids . . . . .FFA

freezing point . . . . .FP

French ethics committee. . . . . CCPRB

frequently asked questions. . . . . FAQ

fresh frozen plasma. . . . . FFP

full blood count . . . . FBC

full of stool / constipated . . . . FOS

full range of movement . . . . FROM

full term. . . . . .FT

full term, normal delivery . . . . FTND

full weight bearing. . . . . .FWB

fully dilated . . . . FD

functional residual capacity. . . . . FRC

functional uterine bleeding . . . . FUB

fundal height . . . . .Fh

A
B
C
D
E
F
G
H
I
J
K
L
M
N
O
P
Q
R
S
T
U
V
W
X
Y
Z

The Institute of Clinical Research

haemoglobin (may also be Hb)	Hgb
haemoglobin (may also be Hgb)	Hb
haemophyllus influenza B	HiB
half life (of a drug)	T1/2
half strength	HS
hand shaking	HS
Hartman's solution	HS
head, eyes, ears, nose, throat	HEENT
headache	H/A
Health Action International	HAI
Health Insurance Portability and Accountability Act (USA)	HIPAA
Health Protection Agency (UK)	HPA
heart attack	HA
heart block	HB
heart rate	HR
heart sounds	HS
heart sounds	S1/S2/S3/S4
hemadsorption (laboratory virus testing)	HAD
hemaglutinin	HA
hemi body irradiation	HBI
hemorrhagic septicemia	HS
Henderson-hasselbach equation (haemoglobin/hematocrit)	H/H
hepatic activity index	HAI
hepatic arterial infusion	HAI
hepatic encephalopathy	HE
hepatitis	Hep
hepatitis A, B virus	HAV; HBV
hepatocellular	HCC
hepatojugular reflex	HJR
hepatosplenomegaly	HSM
hereditary elliptocytosis	HE
hereditary erythrocytosis	HE
hereditary nonpolyposis colorectal cancer	HNPCC
hereditary prostate cancer	HPC
hereditary spherocytosis	HS

H
I

The
Institute
of
Clinical
Research

idiopathic thrombocytopaenic purpura	ITP
if necessary	SOS
immediately	stat
immunoglobulin	Ig
impression/diagnosis	IMP
in vitro fertilisation	IVF
incision and drainage	I+D
incomplete bilateral bundle branch block	IBBBB
incomplete heart block	IHD
incomplete left bundle branch block	ILBBB
incomplete right bundle branch block	IRBBB
increased intraocular tension	T+
IND application form (USA)	FDA 1571
independent ethics committee	IEC
independent review board	IRB
individual quality of life questionnaire	IQoL
infectious disease	ID
inferior	INF
inferior vena cava	IVC
inflammatory bowel disease	IBD
Information Officers in the Pharmaceutical Industry	PIPA
informed consent	IC
infusion	I
in-patient	IP
insertion and removal	I+R
inside diameter	ID
Institute of Clinical Research	ICR
institutional review board	IRB
instructions for use	IFU
insulin dependent diabetes mellitus (Type 1)	IDDM
insulin resistant diabetes mellitus	IRDM
insulin tolerance test	ITT
intake and output	I&O; I/O; I+O
intensive care unit	ICU
intensive therapy unit	ITU

The Institute of Clinical Research

The
Institute
of
Clinical
Research

last patient in	LPI
last patient out	LPO
lateral	lat
laxative	lax
lead	Pb
left	_L
left anterior descending	LAD
left anterior descending coronary artery	LAD
left anterior hemi block	LAHB
left atrial enlargement	LAE
left axis deviation	LAD
left bundle branch block	LBBB
left coronary artery	LCA
left front anterior	LFA
left hypertophia	LHT
left iliac fossa	LIF
left inguinal hernia	LIH
left intercostals space	LICS
left Lateral gaze	LLG
left lower extremity	LLE
left lower lobe	LLL
left lower quadrant	LLQ
left occipital posterior	LOT
left occiput anterior	LOA
left otitis media	LOM
left sternal border	LSB
left upper quadrant	LUQ
left ventricular and diastolic pressure	LVEDP
left ventricular failure	LVF
left ventricular hypertrophy	LVH
length of stay	LOS
lentigo maligna melanoma	LMM
lethal dose	LD
letter of agreement	LOA
leukocytes	leuc

Licensed Practice Nurse	LPN
ligament	Lig
light touch	LT
liquid	Liq
litres per minute	L/min
liver function tests	LFT
liver; kidney right, left; spleen	LKKS
living and well	L&W
local anaesthesia	LA
Local Research Ethics Committee	LREC
locomotor system	LS
long-acting thyroid stimulator	LATS
loss of consciousness / level of consciousness	LOC
low birth weight	LBW
low density lipoproteins	LDL
low flap	LF
low forceps	LF
lower back pain	LBP
lower extremities	LE
lower lid	LL
lower respiratory tract infection	LRTI
lower right quadrant	LRQ
lower segment caesarean section	LSCS
lumbar puncture	LP
lumbar vertebrae/nerves 1st, 2nd	L1, L2 etc
lung function tests	LFT
lupus erythematosus	LE
lutenising hormone	LH
lymphocytes	Lymphs
magnetic resonance angiography	MRA
magnetic resonance imaging	MRI
manipulation under anaesthetic	MUA
manufacturers licence exemption	MLX
Marketing Authorisation	MA

The Institute of Clinical Research

---

memorandum of understanding	MOU
metacarpal	MC
metacarpo-phalangeal joint	MCPJ
metastases	METS
metatarsal	MT
metatarsophalangeal joint	MTPJ
methicillin resistant staphylococcus aureus	MRSA
microbiology advisory committee	MAC
microscopy, culture and sensitivity	M; C&S
microvascular decompression	MVD
midstream specimen of urine; midstream urine	MSSU; MSU
milli-equivalent	mEq
millilitre	Ml
millimetre	Mm
millimetre of mercury (measuring blood pressure)	mmHg
millimole (milliosmole/mosmol)	mMOL
mini mental state examination	MMSE
minimum concentration of drug	C_{min}
minimum inhibitory concentration	MIC
minimum lethal dose	MLD
Ministry of Health (UK)	MOH
Ministry of Health and Welfare (Japan)	MHW
mitral regurgitation	MR
mitral stenosis	MS
monitor's trip report	MTR
monoamine oxidase inhibitor	MAOI
Monthly Index of Medical Specialties	MIMS
morning	mane
morning dose	AM
motor neurone disease	MND
motor vehicle accident	MVA
Multicentre Research Ethics Committee	MREC
multi infarct dementia	MID
multigated cardiac scan (nuclear isotope)	MUGA
multiple endocrine neoplasia	MEN

The Institute of Clinical Research

multiple sclerosis .... MS
multivariate analysis of variance............................ MANOVA
mutual recognition agreement .... MRA
myocardial infarction .... MI

naso-gastric .... NG
National Cancer Research Network (UK) .... NCRN
National Drugs Advisory Board .... NDAB
National Health and Research Council (Australia) .... NH MRC
National Health Service (UK) .... NHS
National Institute of Health (USA) .... NIH
National Patient Safety Agency (UK) .... NPSA
National Physical Laboratory (UK)............................ NPL
nausea and vomiting............................... N&V; N/V
NDA application form (USA)............................ FDA 356
neck of femur .... NOF
neck of humerus.. NOH
neonatal intensive care unit................................... NICU
new active substance .... NAS
new chemical entity.. NCE
new drug application (USA) .... NDA
new molecular entity... NME
NHS Strategic Tracing Service (UK) .... NSTS
night & morning.. N&M
nightly .... Nocté
nil by mouth .... NBM
nitroglycerin .... TNG
no action indicated .... NAI
no active disease .... NAD
no births, one abortion PO,AB1
no carbon required... NCR
no enlargement of liver, kidney, spleen or other
    palpable masses................................... °LKKS/masses
no evidence of recurrence .... NER

no evidence of recurrent disease.................................... NED
no further appointment .... NFA
no jaundice, clubbing, cyanosis, lymphadenopathy, anaemia .... °JCCLA
no known allergies... NKA
no observable effect level .... NOEL
no regular medicines... NRM
non smoker .... NS
non-esterified fatty acids .... NEFA
non-evasive blood pressure .... NBP
non-insulin dependent diabetes mellitus (Type 2) .... NIDDM
non-protein nitrogen... NPN
non-small cell lung carcinoma .... NSCLC
non-specific urethritis.. NSU
non-steroidal anti-inflammatory drug................................ NSAID
non-ulcer dyspepsia .... NUD
Nordic Clinical Data Management (Association) .... NCDM
normal .... N or _N
normal saline .... N/S
normal temperature pressure .... NTP
nose & throat .... N&T
not applicable .... NA
not done .... ND
not known.. NK
not significant.. NS
nothing abnormal discovered .... NAD
nothing by mouth .... NPO
nuclear isotope scan (technetium/sestamibi) .... MIBI
nuclear magnetic resonance (imaging) .... NMR
null hypothesis (statistical term)................................... H°

obsessive compulsive disorder.. OCD
obstetrics & gynaecology .... OBGYN
obstetrics and gynaecology .... Obs Gyn
obstructive sleep apnoea syndrome .... OSAS

A
B
C
D
E
F
G
H
I
J
K
L
M
N
O
P
Q
R
S
T
U
V
W
X
Y
Z

The Institute of Clinical Research

The
Institute
of
Clinical
Research

postoperative day	pod
potassium	K; K$^+$
pounds per square inch	Psi
powder	Pdr
pre-eclampsic toxaemia	PET
pregnancy at term	PAT
pregnant mare's serum gonadotrophin	PMSG
premature atrial, auricular contraction	PAC
premature ventricular contraction	PVC
pre-menstrual tension	PMT
prescribe/prescription/treatment	Rx
prescription	FP10
prescription only medicine	POM
present illness	PI
presenting complaint	PC; P/C
primary biliary cirrhosis	PBC
Primary Care Trust (UK)	PCT
Principal Investigator	PI
prior births; paraplegic	Para
prior to admission	PTA
product licence	PL
product licence application	PLA
product of conception	POC
prognosis	Px
progressive spinal muscular atrophy	PSMA
prolactin (luteotrophic, lactogenic hormone)	LTH
protein bound iodine	PBI
prothrombin time	PT
proximal	prox
proximal interphalangeal (joint)	PIP(J)
pulmonary artery pressure	PAP
pulmonary artery systolic pressure	PAS
pulmonary artery wedge pressure	PAWP
pulmonary embolism	PE
pulmonary function tests	PFTs

pulmonary insufficiency . . . . PI
pulmonary stenosis . . . . PS
pulse rate . . . . PR
pupils equal and reactive to light and accommodation . . . . PERLA
purified protein derivative . . . . PPD
pyrexia of unknown origin . . . . PUO

Qualified Person . . . . QP
quality-adjusted life year . . . . QALY
quality assurance (unit) . . . . QA(U)
quality control . . . . QC
quality control department . . . . QCD
quality management system . . . . QMS
quality of life . . . . QL
quality of life . . . . QOL
quality of life index . . . . QLI
quality of life questionnaire . . . . QOLQ
quality of life score . . . . QLS
quality of well-being . . . . QWB
quality point of service . . . . QPOS
quality-adjusted life expectancy . . . . QALE
quality-adjusted survival . . . . QAS
quick and early diagnosis . . . . QED
quinidine effect . . . . QE

radial pulse . . . . RP
Radiation Protection Officer . . . . RPO
radioallergosorbent test . . . . RAST
radioimmunoassay . . . . RIA
radiotherapy . . . . RT
radioulnar joint . . . . RUJ
raised intracranial pressure . . . . RICP
randomised clinical trial . . . . RCT

The Institute of Clinical Research

A
B
C
D
E
F
G
H
I
J
K
L
M
N
O
P
Q
R
S
T
U
V
W
X
Y
Z

right lower quadrant (abdominal)	RLQ
right upper quadrant	RUQ
right ventricular failure	RVF
risk assessment of drugs – analysis and response	RADAR
road traffic accident	RTA
routine admission	RA
sacral vertebrae/nerves 1st, 2nd	S1, S2 etc

sacro-illiac joint	SIJ
Salivary Immunoreactive Insulin	SIRI
salpingo oophorectomy	S&O
sclerae and conjunctive	S&C
screening and evaluation	S&E
seasonal affective disorder	SAD
second under defined conditions)	KAT
secondary acute non lymphoid leukemia	S-Anill
secondary adhd	S-ADHD
seen by	S/B
self-report data	S DATA
senile dementia Alzheimer type	SDAT
Senior House Officer	SHO
Senior Registrar	SR
sensation	Sen
serious adverse device event	SADE
serious adverse event	SAE
serious adverse reaction	SAR
serious unexpected adverse event	SUA
serious unexpected event	SUE
serum creatinine	SCr
serum gamma-glutamyl transpeptidase	SGGT
serum glutamic-oxaloacetic transaminase	SGOT
serum glutamic-pyruvic transaminase	SGPT
shortness of breath	SOB
shortness of breath at rest	SOBAR

The Institute of Clinical Research

The
Institute
of
Clinical
Research

The
Institute
of
Clinical
Research

ulcerative colitis	UC
ultrasound gall bladder	USGB
ultrasound scan	US; USS
ultraviolet	UV
unavailable	UA
unknown	Ukn
upper respiratory tract infection	URTI
urea and electrolytes	U&E
urinary tract infection	UTI
uro-genital system	UGS

vaccine	VAX
vaccine adverse event reporting system (FDA)	VAERS
vaginal birth after caesarean	VBAC
vaginal delivery	VD
vaginal examination	VE
vaginally	vag
vagotomy and pyloroplasty	V&P
valproic acid	VPA
vancomycin resistant enterococci	VRE
vanillylmandelic acid	VMA
vanilmandelic acid	VMA
variant Creutzfeldt-Jakob disease	vCJD
variant of Avian Flu	H5N1
varicose veins	VV
vascular dementia	VD
vasoactive intestinal peptide	VIP
vastus medialis	VM
venereal disease	VD
venereal diseases research laboratory	VDRL
venous	VEN
venous blood gas	VBG
venous thromboembolic events	V
ventilation/perfusion	

ward round . . . . WR
well developed; well nourished . . . . WDWN
white blood corpuscle . . . . WBC
white cell count (diff = differential) . . . . WCC
with . . . . c; i/c
with European Union member state national statutes and regulations) . . . CA
within normal limits . . . . WNL
Wolff-Parkinson-white (syndrome) . . . . WPW
World Health Organization . . . . WHO
write on label . . . . Sig

x-ray . . . . XR

years old . . . . Y/O

zephiran trisodium phosphate . . . . Z-TSP
zero defects . . . . Z/D
zeta erythrocyte sedimentation rate . . . . Z-ESR
zig zag deoxyribonucleic acid . . . . Z-DNA
Zollinger-Ellison syndrome . . . . ZE